Easing Anxiety and Stress Naturally

A natural, drugless
program to ease stress,
nervous tension and
emotional disturbance

Susan M. Lark, M.D.

Keats Publishing, Inc. 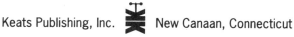 New Canaan, Connecticut

Easing Anxiety and Stress Naturally is not intended as medical advice. Its intent is solely informational and educational. Please consult a health professional should the need for one be indicated.

EASING ANXIETY AND STRESS NATURALLY

This book is excerpted from *Anxiety & Stress*, copyright © 1993 by Susan M. Lark, M.D., and is published by arrangement with Westchester Publishing Company.

ISBN: 0-87983-728-4

Printed in the United States of America

Good Health Guides are published by
Keats Publishing, Inc.
27 Pine Street (Box 876)
New Canaan, Connecticut 06840-0876

Contents

INTRODUCTION

Emotional symptoms due to excessive life stresses are very common and affect millions of women in our society from preadolescence to the postmenopausal years. Upset feelings created by stress can trigger nervous tension, irritability and edginess. In extreme cases, women will react with feelings of anxiety, sometimes expressed in episodes of fear and panic. Unpleasant physical symptoms such as rapid heart beat and shortness of breath may then be triggered, leaving a woman's physical body feeling as upset and out of control as her emotions. Anxiety can impede a woman's ability to function optimally in the workplace, at home and with co-workers, friends and family. In fact, 10 percent of the American population—between 20 and 30 million people—suffer from anxiety symptoms each year.

Emotional symptoms of stress stem from a broad range of emotional, social, chemical and physical imbalances. Some women have anxiety episodes that are emotionally based in childhood upsets and traumas, while others may develop stress symptoms after severe life crises such as a death, divorce or job loss. Anxiety can also be a primary symptom of such medical problems as PMS, transition into menopause, hyperthyroidism and hypoglycemia. And anxiety can arise from nutritional deficiencies as well as the improper use of drugs or alcohol.

Historically, women with anxiety have been treated with drug therapies, sometimes combined with counseling or psychotherapy. Though antianxiety drugs help relieve the emotional symptoms, they can be a mixed blessing. Often they produce unpleasant side effects as well as psychological and physical dependence. Counseling may be ineffective if the underlying physical causes are not diagnosed or are ignored. Many women have told me of their fruitless search for adequate relief as they went from physician to physician, trying different combinations of medications.

What is missing from this scenario is the woman's participation in her own healing process. In my experience, women can reap tremendous benefits from practicing anxiety-relieving self-help techniques. These techniques, which encompass specific principles of diet, nutrition, exercise and stress management, can often replace medication. Even in more severe cases, the use of self-help techniques along with medication produces better results than medication alone. In addition, the practice of self-help techniques can help women reduce not only their dependence on medication, but the likelihood of recurring symptoms.

Over the past 20 years, I have researched the use of diet, nutrition and many other lifestyle techniques to treat my patients' problems of anxiety and stress. Specific acupressure points, yoga stretches and exercise routines, as well as many other stress management techniques, offer a wide variety of self-care options. I have been delighted when my patients find these self-help treatments so beneficial and effective.

HOW TO USE THIS BOOK

My purpose in writing this book is to share with women the self-care techniques that I have found to be most useful through many years of medical practice. The anxiety and stress self-help program is written so that each reader can select from a wide variety of treatment options, including diet, nutrition, vitamins, minerals and herbs, programs of stress reduction, physical exercise, acupressure massage, deep breathing exercises and yoga stretches. By overlapping treatments from various disciplines, most women are able to put together a highly effective individualized treatment plan.

Read through the entire book first to familiarize yourself with the material. Then make a monthly calendar (page 13) to help you evaluate your symptoms and chart your risk factors and stress-creating lifestyle habits. Try all the therapies; some will probably make you feel better than others. Establish a regimen that works for you and use it every day.

This anxiety and stress self-help program is practical and easy to follow either by itself or in conjunction with a medical or therapeutic program. This book can help many women reduce the severity of symptoms and prevent recurrence of the disease process. You can experience a feeling of wellness with a self-help program that will radiate out and touch your whole life. Just like my patients, you may positively transform your life by following these beneficial self-help techniques.

WHAT IS ANXIETY?

Anxiety is described as "a state of being uneasy, apprehensive or worried about what may happen" or a "feeling of being powerless and unable to cope with threatening events . . . [characterized] by physical tension." We all encounter everyday, real-life situations to which anxiety is a reasonable response. They can be as major as a death, divorce or job loss or as seemingly minor as going to the doctor or meeting new people at a social event. Anxiety can vary in intensity from being an appropriate response to stressful or difficult situations to being a psychiatric disorder.

While most women experience anxiety emotionally as upset and distress, we also react to these feelings on a physical level. An alarm reaction is set off called the "fight-or-flight" response. This is a powerful protective mechanism that allows our body to mobilize energy quickly and either escape from or confront any type of danger. This response occurs to any perceived threat, whether it is physically real, psychologically upsetting or imaginary. Even our thoughts and feelings can trigger this response.

The flight-or-fight response begins in our nervous system, which consists of the brain, the spinal cord and the peripheral nerves. It is divided by function into two parts: the voluntary nervous system and autonomic nervous system. The voluntary nervous system manages conscious activity. For example, if you place your hand on a hot stove, the brain immediately tells you to move it away fast before you burn yourself. The autonomic nervous system regulates unconscious functions, such as muscle tension, pulse rate, respiration, glandular function and the circulation of the blood. A flight-or fight response stimulates the autonomic nervous system, triggering several different physical responses. For instance, the adrenal glands increase their output of adrenaline and cortisone, which causes the heart and pulse rate to speed up, breathing to become shallow and rapid, hands and feet to become icy cold and muscles to tighten up and become tense and contracted.

Though our physiological response to anxiety or stress is the same no matter what the initial stressor—physical danger, psychological distress or imaginary threat—the chemical trigger for anxiety can vary greatly. In women with anxiety or panic episodes, the sympathetic nervous system is too often in a state of readiness. This puts them in a constant state of fight-or-flight.

Any of four body systems may be compromised with anxiety: (1) The *nervous system*, which consists of fibers connecting the brain, organs and muscles that transmit impulses allowing normal bodily sensation, movement and the experience and expression of moods and feelings. (2) The *endocrine or glandular system*, which regulates reproductive and metabolic functions by secreting chemicals (hormones) into the bloodstream that carry messages from one gland to another. (3) The *immune system*, which fights foreign invaders such as bacteria, viruses and cancer cells. (4) The *cardiovascular system*, which consists of the heart and all the blood vessels in the body.

TYPES OF ANXIETY DISORDERS

Women experience three major types of psychologically based anxiety disorders: generalized anxiety disorder, panic disorder and phobias. Research in brain chemistry has shown that these disorders may also be linked to specific chemical changes in the brain, thus suggesting a strong mind-body link. The field of psychiatry recognizes other types of anxiety disorders, such as obsessive-compulsive disorder and post-traumatic stress syndrome, which will not be covered in this book.

Generalized Anxiety Disorder
This is characterized by chronic anxiety (of at least 6 months duration) that is focused on real-life issues, such as problems with work, finances, relationships or health, which feel dangerous or threatening to a woman's security and well-being. These issues often elicit deeper emotional concerns, such as fear of abandonment, rejection or not being loved (which may underlie troubled personal relationships), fear of failure, inability to cope effectively with stressful situations and even fear of death when there are health concerns. Common symptoms include frequent upset, worry and nervous tension, as well as insomnia, irritability, difficulty concentrating and startling easily. Physical symptoms include typical fight-or-flight responses: rapid heartbeat, cold hands and feet, shortness of breath, muscle tension, shakiness, depression and chronic fatigue.

The disorder, which can date back to childhood, but is most often diagnosed in the twenties or thirties, occurs with equal frequency among men and women. If you suffer from generalized anxiety disorder, consult a physician to rule out any possible medical disorders, such as hyperthyroidism, food allergies or PMS that could be mistaken for an anxiety disorder. In addition, since anxiety and depression can coexist, it is important to know which is the primary, as treatment will differ.

Panic Disorder
Panic is characterized by the sudden onset of intense fear that occurs unexpectedly for no apparent reason. The acute phase lasts only a few minutes, though symptoms may persist at a lesser intensity. For this diagnosis, a woman must have at least four panic attacks in one month or significant worry throughout an entire month following one panic attack. As in generalized anxiety disorder, the symptoms are typical of the fight-or-flight reaction, although much more intense and disabling. They include at least four of the following: rapid heartbeat or heart palpitations, chest pain, shakiness, dizziness, faintness, shortness of breath, cold hands and feet, numbness and tingling in the hands and feet, intestinal distress, sweating, feelings of losing control and feelings of unreality. Between panic episodes, women tend to worry excessively about their recurrence.

Panic disorder tends to coexist with agoraphobia (fear of open spaces or public places), which affects 5 percent of the U.S. population; only 1 percent suffering from panic disorder alone. Panic disorder tends to develop during the twenties. It is important to differentiate panic disorder from medical problems such as mitral valve prolapse (which can coexist with panic disorder and produce similar symptoms), hypoglycemia or chemical imbalances like drug withdrawal or excessive caffeine intake.

Phobias
Phobias are characterized by an excessive, persistent and often irrational fear of a person, object, place or situation. The person will postpone or avoid facing situations that trigger the phobia, such as being in public places or going to social gatherings or the doctor, which can compromise day-to-day functioning or even one's health and well-being.

Agoraphobia (fear of open or public spaces) is the most common of all anxiety disorders, and three-quarters of all agoraphobics are women. Their overriding fear is of being trapped in a place—bus, department store, tunnel—where escape is difficult and of being overcome by a panic attack. As the phobia worsens, even thinking about being in a situation can engender panic, so they often restrict their range of activities and locations. Luckily, a combination of medication, counseling and stress management training will produce good results in as many as 90 percent of all people suffering from this condition.

Social phobia is another common form, which occurs when there is fear of performing in front of other people or being scrutinized by other people. Common social phobias include fear of public speaking, eating in public, being watched or looked at while at social gatherings or being photographed in a crowded room. This phobia may begin in a shy child and can persist throughout adult life (although severity of social phobias tends to decrease with age). Many people employ a variety of effective self-help techniques to deal with social phobias. Classes on self-image and self-esteem use a variety of techniques, and some women find one-on-one counseling very effective.

A third type of phobia, called simple phobia, involves fear of a particular situation or object. Common examples include fear of animals (dogs or snakes), airplanes (fear they will crash), heights or even having blood drawn for testing. Many simple phobias originate in childhood and persist into adult life (though the adult may recognize they are irrational), or they are triggered by a traumatic event, such as being stuck in an elevator. Simple phobias are easiest to treat. The fear response can usually be lessened by gradual exposure to the phobia-inducing situation or by practicing a variety of stress-reducing techniques such as affirmations (discussed in the stress-reduction section of this book).

RISK FACTORS FOR ANXIETY DISORDERS

• **Physiological Imbalances:** Research suggests that women with generalized anxiety disorder may have an imbalance of gamma amino butyric acid (GABA), a neurotransmitter in their brain. While the mechanism triggering generalized anxiety is not known, people's anxiety diminishes when they are given GABA or drugs that increase GABA activity.

• **Genetic Factors:** While 5 percent of the entire population suffers from agoraphobia, the rate of agoraphobia in people with one diagnosed parent is 15 to 25 percent. Rates for identical and fraternal twins are also higher.

• **Family Programming:** Parents who are critical perfectionists, who have phobias, who are overly controlling and suppress a child's self-assertiveness seem to produce insecurity, fear and dependency in susceptible children. However, not all children raised in such environments develop anxiety disorders. The likelihood is greater in children born with more sensitive, reactive personalities whose fight-or-flight response is easily triggered.

• **Major Long- and Short-Term Life Stresses:** Women who have suffered from major life stresses over a long period of time, such as marriage to an abusive husband, chronic illness in family members or constant financial worries, may find it difficult to handle stress. Quick significant life change or dislocation—such as death of a spouse or even positive events like marriage—can also produce anxiety.

• **Personal Belief Systems:** Many women have belief systems—poor self-image, low self-esteem or a negative view of the world—that lead to anxiety disorders, and they may be consumed by fearful self-talk.

PHYSICAL CONDITIONS ASSOCIATED WITH ANXIETY

Solutions to the following physical conditions will be discussed later in the book.

• **Premenstrual Syndrome (PMS):** More than 90 percent of women with PMS in my practice complain of heightened anxiety and irritability that increases in intensity the week or two prior to menstruation (along with more than 150 physical symptoms. For many women, the emotional symptoms and fatigue are the most severe, adversely affecting family relationships and their ability to work. PMS affects one-third to one-half of American women between the ages of 20 and 50 (most severely in their 30s and 40s), or as many as 10 to 14 million women. More than 24 hormonal and chemical imbalances can trigger PMS symptoms; many factors increase the risk of PMS in susceptible women.

• **Menopause:** The end of all menstrual bleeding occurs between the ages of 48 and 52 for most women. The transition to menopause takes place gradually (over four to six years), triggered by a slowdown in the estrogen production of the ovaries. Anxiety, mood swings, irregular bleeding, hot flashes and fatigue often accompany this process in 80 percent of menopausal women.

• **Hyperthyroidism:** When the thyroid gland excretes an excessive amount of thyroid hormone, hyperthyroidism (Graves disease) occurs. Symptoms of hyperthyroidism can mimic those of anxiety attacks, including generalized anxiety, insomnia, easy fatigability and rapid heartbeat. Other symptoms, such as weight loss despite a ravenous appetite, quick movements, trembling hands, difficulty focusing the eyes and an enlarged thyroid, should tip off both the woman and her physician of the imbalance. Hyperthyroidism should always be considered when diagnosing the cause of anxiety.

Hypoglycemia: Glucose, or sugar, is the major fuel our bodies run on. When blood sugar levels fall too low, people experience many symptoms of hypoglycemia similar to those of anxiety attacks, including anxiety, irritability, trembling, disorientation, light-headedness, spaciness and even palpitations. Women who eat a diet high in simple sugars which trigger hypoglycemia often feel as though they are on an emotional roller coaster, tossed from highs of anxiety and irritability to lows of fatigue and depression.

• **Immune System Imbalances: Allergies, Including Food Allergies:** Allergic reactions can cause mood changes such as anxiety. Allergies occur when the body's immune system, which fights off invaders such as viruses, bacteria, overreacts to harmless substances—typically pollens, molds or foods. Common food allergens include wheat, milk (and milk products), alcohol, chocolate, eggs, yeast, peanuts, citrus fruits, tomatoes, corn and shellfish. Some allergic reactions are easily diagnosed because wheezing, itching and tearing of the eyes, nasal congestion and hives occur immediately upon contact. Some allergic reactions are delayed, including anxiety, depression, fatigue, dizziness, spaciness, head-aches, joint aches and pains and eczema. The person may be unaware that an allergy is causing the symptoms. Often, you crave the foods that you are allergic to; common cravings are chocolate, chips, pasta, bread and milk products. Food allergies tend to be worse during the premenstrual time. There are many tests for allergies (consult your health practitioner) or try a low-stress elimination diet you can do yourself.

• **Cardiovascular System Disorders: Mitral Valve Prolapse:** This heart condition can cause anxiety-like episodes of palpitations, chest pain, shortness of breath and fatigue. It appears to be present more frequently in people with anxiety and panic episodes than in the general population. Undue stress and stimulants such as caffeine-containing beverages like coffee, tea and colas should be eliminated to avoid triggering episodes. Taking supplements of calcium, magnesium and potassium help regulate and reduce cardiac irritability.

EVALUATING YOUR SYMPTOMS

I have found over the years that a woman's own evaluation of her symptoms is as important as the actual treatments. Begin by making a monthly calendar of your symptoms (photocopy the one on page 13) and rate their severity, starting today. Then read over the next section on risk factors and evaluations to see which of your habits are contributing to your health problems. This will make it easier to pick specific treatments for your symptoms and devise a personal treatment program as outlined in the later self-help sections of the book. After that, you may want to keep making monthly calendars to check your progress.

RISK FACTORS

You are at higher risk for developing symptoms of anxiety and stress if you have any of the risk factors listed below. Make a list of the risk factors that apply to you.

Relatives with a history of anxiety disorders, phobias or agoraphobia
History of overly critical parents, lack of emotional nurturing
History of parents who suppressed and punished communication and verbalization of feelings
History of fearful and overly cautious parents
Childhood history of fearing separation from parents (going to school, play activities or even falling asleep without parents)
Significant life stress such as death, illness or divorce preceding onset of excessive anxiety
PMS
Menopause
Hyperthyroidism (excessive thyroid function)
Hypoglycemia

Monthly Calendar of Anxiety Symptoms

Grade your symptoms as you experience them each month.
○ None　✓ Mild　◗ Moderate　● Severe

Month

DAY OF MONTH	1	2	3	4	5	6	7	8	9	10	11	12	13	14	15	16	17	18	19	20	21	22	23	24	25	26	27	28	29	30	31
SYMPTOM																															
Excessive tension or nervousness																															
Feelings of being on edge																															
Easily startled, jumpy																															
Difficulty falling or staying asleep																															
Easily angered, irritable																															
Restlessness, easily excited																															
Dizziness, shakiness, tremulousness																															
Difficulty concentrating or focusing																															
Blue moods alternating with anxiety																															
Excessive tiredness or fatigue																															
Fear of certain locations, situations																															
Fear of other people																															
Frequent nightmares																															
Muscle tightness or tension																															
Fast or irregular heartbeat																															
Chest pain																															
Shortness of breath																															
Excessive sweating																															
Dry mouth																															
Intestinal cramps, nausea, diarrhea																															
Frequent urination																															
Hot flashes or feeling of chilliness																															
Cold hands and feet																															
Tightness in throat or lump in throat																															

Food allergies or allergy to food additives (such as Nutrasweet)
Food addictions
Mitral valve prolapse
Use of estrogen-containing medication
Withdrawal from alcohol, tranquilizers or sedatives
Use of recreational drugs (such as cocaine, amphetamines) that increase anxiety levels
Excessive use of coffee, black tea, colas, chocolates or other caffeine-containing foods
Excessive use of sugar
Calcium, magnesium or potassium deficiency
Lack of B vitamins

Eating Habits Evaluation

All foods listed below as high-stress foods can worsen anxiety. If you eat a number of them, or if you eat any of them frequently, your nutritional habits may be significantly contributing to your symptoms. All the foods listed under high-nutrient, low-stress foods may help relieve or prevent symptoms of anxiety. Include them frequently in your diet.

Make a list of the foods you eat and the frequency with which you eat them: never, once a month, once a week, twice a week or more.

High-Stress Foods

Cow's milk	Wheat-based flour
Cow's cheese	Pastries
Butter	Added salt
Ice cream	Bouillon
Eggs	Commercial
Chocolate	salad dressing
Sugar	Catsup
Alcohol	Coffee
Beef	Black tea
Pork	Soft drinks
Lamb	Hot dogs
Wheat bread	Ham
Wheat noodles	Bacon

High-Nutrient, Low-Stress Foods

Avocado	Radishes	Raw filberts
Beans	Spinach	Raw pecans
Broccoli	Squash	Raw walnuts

Brussels sprouts
Cabbage
Carrots
Celery
Collards
Cucumbers
Eggplant
Garlic
Horseradish
Kale
Lettuce
Mustard greens
Okra
Onions
Parsnips
Peas
Potatoes

Sweet potatoes
Tomatoes
Turnips
Turnip greens
Yams
Brown rice
Millet
Barley
Oatmeal
Buckwheat
Rye
Corn
Raw flax seeds
Raw pumpkin seeds
Raw sesame seeds
Raw sunflower seeds
Raw almonds

Apples
Bananas
Berries
Pears
Seasonal fruits
Corn oil
Flax oil
Olive oil
Sesame oil
Safflower oil
Poultry
Fish

Exercise Habits

Exercise helps relieve symptoms of anxiety and reduce symptoms of muscular tension accompanying emotional distress. All people need at least three exercise periods per week. However, some women with anxiety tend to overexercise, actually triggering panic symptoms; they should modify their current regimen.

Make a list of the frequency with which you do any of the following: never, once a month, once or twice a week, three times a week or more.

Jogging
Walking
Bicycling
Skiing
Swimming
Aerobic dancing
Jumping rope
Ice skating

Roller skating
Baseball
Handball
Racquetball
Tennis
Soccer
Basketball
Weight lifting

Bowling
Table tennis
Golf
Croquet
Yoga
Stretching
Gardening

If the symptoms of lack of physical fitness and stamina listed below pertain to you, it's best to start a physical fitness program slowly and gradually until your body is more accustomed to exercise. Then design an exercise regimen with your physician.

Fatigue, tiredness, lethargy
Tiredness or exhaustion when walking less than a mile

Shortness of breath when walking less than a mile
Tiredness or exhaustion when walking up a flight of stairs
Shortness of breath when walking up a flight of stairs
Excessive weight or obesity
Poor muscle tone
Excessive muscle tension and/or cramping during physical activity
Eyestrain
Chronic neck pain and muscle tension
Chronic shoulder and upper-middle-back tension
Grinding of teeth (bruxism)
Chronic low back pain
Chronic abdominal tension
Chronic arm tension

Daily Exercise Diary

Make a daily exercise diary listing the following points: date, time, exercise type, session length, pulse rate, emotional responses and physical responses. Keeping this diary will help you determine if your current exercise program is appropriate for helping to reduce your anxiety symptoms as well as promoting optimal physical conditioning. A good exercise program should leave you feeling energized and relaxed at all times. Be sure to do activities you enjoy so you look forward to them. If, after filling out the diary, you find your exercise program is not satisfactory, then switch or add other activities.

When doing vigorous aerobic exercise, make sure that the session increases your pulse rate to the optimal range for your age:

Age	Pulse rate (also indicates heart rate)
20–29	145–164
30–39	130–156
40–49	130–148
50–59	122–140
60–69+	116–132

Stress Evaluation Tool

If you are experiencing any of the following life events, list those that apply to you.

Death of spouse or close family member
Divorce from spouse
Death of a close friend

Legal separation from spouse
Loss of job
Radical loss of financial security
Major personal injury or illness (gynecologic or other cause)
Future surgery for gynecologic or other illness
Beginning a new marriage
Foreclosure of mortgage or loan
Lawsuit lodged against you
Marriage reconciliation
Change in health of a family member
Major trouble with boss or co-workers
Increase in responsibility—at job or home
Sexual harassment, rape or wife battering
Learning you are pregnant
Difficulties with your sexual abilities
Gaining a new family member
Change to a different job
Increase in number of marital arguments
New loan or mortgage of more than $100,000
Son or daughter leaving home
Major disagreement with in-laws or friends
Spouse begins or stops work
Recognition for outstanding achievements
Begin or end education
Undergo a change in living conditions
Revise or alter your personal habits
Change in work hours or conditions
Change of residence
Change in church or club activities
Change in social activities
Change in sleeping habits
Changing diet or eating habits
You go on vacation
The year-end holidays occur

Listing many items in the first third of this scale indicates major life stress and possible vulnerability to serious illness. The more items listed in the first two-thirds, the higher your stress quotient. Do everything possible to manage your stress in a healthy way. Eat the foods that provide a high-nutrient, low-stress diet, exercise on a regular basis and learn methods of stress reduction and deep breathing.

If you list fewer items, you are probably at lower risk for illness. Because stresses too minimal to include in this evaluation may also play a part in increasing your anxiety, you will still benefit from practicing stress reduction techniques. Stress management is very important in helping you gain control over muscle tension.

Daily Stress Evaluation

Not all stresses have a major impact on our lives; most of us experience a multitude of small life stresses on a daily basis. The effects of these stresses are cumulative and can trigger chronic wear and tear on our immune, endocrine and circulatory systems. However, these stresses can trigger major upsets in some women with severe anxiety. List each item that applies to you.

Work
• Too much responsibility. Too many demands made on you. You worry about getting all your work done and doing it well.
• Time urgency. You always feel rushed. There are not enough hours in the day to complete your work.
• Job instability. There are layoffs at your company and much insecurity and concern among your fellow employees.
• Job performance. You don't feel that you are working up to your maximum capability because of outside stresses. You are un-happy with your performance and worried about job security.
• Difficulty getting along with boss and co-workers. Your boss is too picky, critical and demanding. You must work closely with difficult co-workers.
• Understimulation. Work is boring and makes you tired. You wish you were somewhere else.
• Uncomfortable physical plant. Lights are too bright or dim; noises are too loud; you are exposed to noxious fumes or chemicals. you find it hard to concentrate with too much activity around you.

Home
• Organization. Home is always messy; chores are half-finished.
• Time. There is too much to do and never enough time to do it all.
• Responsibility. Too many demands are made on you. You need more help.

Spouse or Significant Other
• Hostile communication. There is too much negative emotion and drama. You are always upset or angry.

• Not enough communications. You both tend to hold in your feelings and not discuss issues. An emotional bond is lacking between you.

• Discrepancy in communications. One person talks about feelings too much, the other person too little.

• Affection. There is not enough holding, touching and loving in your relationship. Or you are uncomfortable by your partner's demands for affection.

• Sexuality. There is not enough sexual intimacy and you feel deprived. Or your partner demands sex too often.

• Children. They make too much noise and too many demands on your time. They are hard to discipline.

• Extended family. Parents, siblings or other relatives are negative, critical, demanding and engage in inappropriate social or addictive behavior. Interactions trigger negative emotional response.

Your Emotional State

• Too much negative self-talk. You constantly worry about every little thing and about what can go wrong.

• Excessive fearfulness of situations. Certain situations or locations trigger fears, such as being on an elevator or eating in a restaurant.

• Excessive fearfulness of public activities. You're afraid of public speaking, being in a social group or going to parties.

• Victimization. Everyone takes advantage of you or wants to hurt you.

• Poor self-image. You are always finding fault with yourself.

• Too critical. You are always finding fault with others rather than seeing their good sides.

• Inability to relax. You are always tense, restless and wound up.

• Not enough self-renewal. You don't play enough or take enough time off to relax and have fun.

• Feelings of depression alternate with anxiety. You feel blue, isolated, tearful and are filled with self-blame and hopelessness. Fatigue and low energy are problems.

• Too angry. Small life issues upset you unduly. You become easily angry and irritable with your husband, children, co-workers or clients.

How many items have you listed? Becoming aware of them is the first step toward lessening their effects on your life.

DIETARY PRINCIPLES

Food selection can play a major role in reducing symptoms. I have seen thousands of women suffering anxiety symptoms due to many different emotional and physical causes improve when they change their diets. And I've seen continuing stressful eating habits actually work against other therapeutic measures. The importance of healthful dietary practices in the treatment of anxiety should not be underestimated.

FOODS TO AVOID

The list of foods that increase anxiety and should be avoided may surprise you. It contains not only junk foods, but foods that are considered staples of the American diet. All of the following foods should be entirely eliminated or at least sharply limited to an occasional treat. Some women may find they need to eliminate anxiety-causing foods gradually; the elimination process itself can cause stress so it should be done gently. Other women find that the cold-turkey approach works best.

Caffeine

Many women with high levels of stress mistakenly use caffeine in coffee, black tea, soft drinks and chocolate to help them get through the day's tasks. However, caffeine triggers anxiety symptoms because it directly stimulates several arousal mechanisms, such as the fight-or-flight response and the release of stress hormones from the adrenal glands. Caffeine also depletes the body's stores of B-complex vitamins and essential minerals, such as potassium, which increases anxiety, mood swings and fatigue.

If you suffer from moderate to severe anxiety symptoms due to any cause, I recommend reducing your caffeine consumption to one cup of coffee (averaging 81 to 146 mg of caffeine) per day and try to eliminate cola drinks (36 to 57 mg), caffeinated tea (29 to 64 mg), cocoa (13 mg) and chocolate candy (4 to 24 mg). Some women may find that eliminating caffeine abruptly causes unpleasant withdrawal symptoms such as headaches, depression and fatigue. In these cases, decrease the amounts slowly over a period of several months, substituting first decaffeinated coffee (4 mg) and finally herbal teas. Many herbal teas, like chamomile, hops and peppermint, reduce anxiety by relaxing the body.

Sugar

Glucose, a simple form of sugar, is the food that provides our body with its main source of energy. A steady supply of glucose helps produce the hundreds of thousands of chemical reactions our body needs to perform its daily functions, with the brain requiring 20 percent of the total glucose available to function optimally. However, the form in which you take glucose into your body can affect your mood in a profound manner.

Unfortunately, many Americans obtain their sugar intake through excess simple sugar—the refined white sugar in most soft drinks, convenience foods and desserts. (Refined white flour in pasta and bread also acts like simple sugar.) With simple sugar so prevalent in many foods, sugar addiction is common and most Americans consume too much sugar—averaging 120 pounds per year. This excessive level of sugar intake can be a major trigger for anxiety symptoms. You may initially feel "high" after eating sugar, and then experience a rapid crash in your energy level. When your blood sugar level falls too low, you begin to feel anxious, jittery, spacey and confused because your brain is deprived of its necessary fuel. Excessive use of sugar has other detrimental effects like depleting the body's B-complex vitamins and minerals (the role of vitamins and minerals is discussed in the next section), thereby increasing nervous tension, anxiety and irritability.

Satisfy your sweet tooth with healthier foods such as fruit or grain-based desserts, like oatmeal cookies sweetened with fruit or honey. Instead of disrupting your mood and energy level, they actually have a healthful and balancing effect.

Alcohol

Women with moderate to severe anxiety and mood swings should avoid alcohol entirely (because it is a simple sugar) or limit its use to occasional small amounts. Like other sugars, excessive use can increase anxiety, which is particularly pronounced in PMS-related hypoglycemia.

The nervous system is particularly susceptible to the negative effects of alcohol. Alcohol can cause profound behavioral and psychological changes in women who use it excessively. Symptoms of emotional upset triggered by alcohol can also promote a tendency toward chronic candida infections. Women with candida-related mood upset and fatigue need to avoid alcohol entirely. Many women with allergies are sensitive to the yeast in alcohol, which worsens their allergic symptoms.

I recommend that women with anxiety symptoms use alcohol very rarely, not exceeding 4 ounces of wine, 12 ounces of beer or 1 ounce of hard liquor per day. Women who are particularly susceptible to the negative effects of alcohol shouldn't drink at all. If you wish, nonalcoholic beverages, such as mineral water with a twist of lime, "near" beer and light wine, are good substitutes.

Food Additives

Several thousand chemical additives, including aspartame (Nutrasweet) used in diet foods, monosodium glutamate (MSG) used in Chinese restaurants and nitrates and nitrites used in cured meats such as hot dogs, bacon and ham produce allergic and anxiety-like symptoms in many people. For instance, I have had patients complain that aspartame precipitated panic-like symptoms, such as rapid heart beat, shallow breathing, headaches, anxiety, spaciness and dizziness. Since it is used in so many processed diet foods, susceptible women need to avoid all low-calorie, sugar-free drinks, jams, desserts and other foods.

Dairy Products

Although dairy products have traditionally been touted as one of the four basic food groups, they are extremely difficult for the body to digest and can worsen depression and fatigue in many women with anxiety symptoms. In addition to many other unhealthy effects, dairy products can intensify allergy symptoms in general, triggering anxiety, mood swings and even fatigue in susceptible women and should therefore be avoided.

Women who have depended on dairy products for their calcium intake naturally wonder what alternative sources to use. There are many other good dietary sources of this essential nutrient, including beans, peas, soybeans, sesame seeds, soup stock made from chicken or fish bones and green leafy vegetables. Soy, potato and nut milks, available in health food stores, are excellent substitutes in food preparation. Use a supplement containing calcium, magnesium and vitamin D to make sure your intake is sufficient.

Red Meats and Poultry

Like dairy products, meat tends to increase depression and fatigue because the extremely dense quality of the protein in meat and a high level of fat make it difficult for the body to digest. Therefore sharply curtail meat consumption. However, if you need to include meat in your diet, chicken with the skin removed and fish are better choices because they are lower in saturated fat content. Vegetables, such as legumes, starches, raw seeds and grains, are other good sources of protein.

Wheat and Other Gluten-Containing Grains

Women who have food allergies or PMS- or menopause-related mood problems may have difficulty digesting wheat. The protein in wheat, called gluten, is highly allergenic and difficult for the body to break down, absorb and assimilate. Women with wheat intolerance are prone to fatigue, depression and digestive symptoms, and wheat consumption can worsen emotional symptoms and fatigue.

No matter what the cause of your anxiety, if your symptoms are severe, you should eliminate wheat from your diet at least for one to three months during the early stages of recovery. Oats and rye, which also contain gluten, should be eliminated initially along with wheat. Although corn and rice do not contain gluten, most women use them so frequently that they build up an intolerance during times of fatigue. The least stressful grain is buckwheat, but also try quinoa and amaranth found in health food stores. As you start to regain emotional equilibrium, you may add rice and corn back into the diet; wait to include wheat, oats and rye until your recovery is complete.

Salt

Although salt does not specifically increase anxiety, women should watch their salt intake carefully and avoid excessive use. Too much salt in the diet can cause many physical problems, including high blood pressure and risk of osteoporosis. Unfortunately, fast foods and most processed, frozen and canned foods contain large amounts of salt. For an antianxiety diet, I recommend eliminating table and cooking salt and using seasonings such as garlic, herbs, spices and lemon juice. Read labels on all foods; if the word *sodium* (salt) appears high on the list of ingredients, don't buy the product.

FOODS THAT HELP RELIEVE ANXIETY

The foods you should eat when anxious, depressed or fatigued should leave you feeling as good as, or better than, you felt before the meal. These foods should support and accelerate the healing process of any illness that underlies the emotional symptoms. Begin to develop an awareness of how your food selections affect your emotional well-being. If a particular food makes you feel anxious, jittery, depressed or fatigued, eliminate it. To achieve these goals, limit your diet initially to low-stress foods, including most vegetables, fruits, starches, nuts and such grains as buckwheat, quinoa, amaranth, corn and rice. As your symptoms diminish, you can eat a wider range of foods, adding more fruits, grains, oils, fish and poultry in moderation.

Vegetables

Vegetables are outstanding foods for stress relief. Many vegetables are high in minerals like calcium, magnesium and potassium, which have been shown to have a relaxant effect and reduce depression. Some of the best sources for these minerals include beet greens, broccoli, kale, mustard greens, spinach and Swiss chard.

Many vegetables are high in vitamin C, an important antistress vitamin which promotes healthy adrenal hormone production. This is particularly important for women with anxiety due to emotional upset or allergies. Vegetables high in vitamin C include broccoli, Brussels sprouts, cauliflower, kale, parsley, peas, peppers, potatoes and tomatoes. Vegetables highest in vitamin A, which helps prevent allergies and infections, are carrots, collards, green onions, kale, parsley, spinach, squash and turnip greens.

Vegetables are easy to digest. Steaming is the best cooking method, because it preserves the essential nutrients. Some women with extreme symptoms may want to puree vegetables in a blender. As you begin to recover, try adding raw foods such as salads, juices and raw vegetables for more texture and variety.

Fruits

Fruits also contain a wide range of nutrients that can relieve anxiety and stress. Like many vegetables, fruits are excellent sources of vitamin C and bioflavonoids, especially berries and melons. Although citrus fruits—oranges, grapefruits—are other good sources, they are highly acidic and difficult for many women with food allergies or sensitive digestive tracts to digest, so it's best to avoid them in the early stages of treatment. Certain fruits—including bananas, blackberries and raisins—are excellent sources of calcium, magnesium and potassium. All fruits, in fact, are excellent sources of potassium.

Fresh fruits are excellent substitutes for foods high in refined white sugar. Although high in sugar, fruit's high fiber content helps slow down absorption, thereby stabilizing blood sugar levels. I recommend that women with anxiety do not consume fruit juices, which act like table sugar and can heighten mood swings.

Starches

Potatoes, sweet potatoes and yams, all good sources of A, B and C vitamins, are soft, well-tolerated complex carbohydrates that provide an additional source of easy-to-digest protein. Like other complex carbohydrates, starches calm the mood by regulating the blood sugar level. You can steam, mash, bake and eat them alone or include them with a variety of vegetables in other low-stress dishes, casseroles and soups.

Legumes

I highly recommend legumes to combat depression and fatigue. Beans and peas are excellent sources of calcium, magnesium, potassium and vitamin B complex. They are also excellent, easily used sources of protein and, when eaten with whole grains, can be substituted for meat at many meals (good combinations are rice and beans and corn bread and split pea soup). Legumes are also an excellent source of fiber, they are digested slowly and can help regulate the blood sugar level.

Some women have gas when they eat beans. You can minimize gas by taking digestive enzymes and eating beans in small quantities. Because legumes contain high levels of protein, women with severe fatigue or digestive problems may find them difficult to digest at first, so I recommend beginning with green beans or peas, lentils, lima beans, split peas, fresh sprouts and possibly tofu. As your energy level improves, add such delicious legumes as black, pinto and kidney beans and chickpeas.

Whole Grains

Although you should eliminate some wheat and other gluten-containing grains when first starting an antianxiety program, many whole grains have tremendous health benefits for women suffering from nervous tension. Whole grains are excellent sources of mood-stabilizing nutrients like vitamin B-complex, vitamin E, many essential minerals, complex carbohydrates, protein, essential fatty acids and fiber. Like legumes, whole grains help stabilize the blood sugar level.

Brown rice and corn are good choices for women with mild to moderate anxiety symptoms, as are buckwheat, quinoa and amaranth. Pasta, cereals, flour and other foods made from these grain alternatives can be purchased in health food stores. Women with allergy-related anxiety symptoms need to rotate a variety of nongluten-containing grains in the diet to prevent anxiety due to allergic reactions or fatigue.

Seeds and Nuts

Seeds and nuts are the best sources of B-complex vitamins, vitamin E and essential fatty acids needed to prevent both the emotional and physical symptoms of PMS, menopause, emotional upsets and allergies. The best sources of both fatty acids are raw flax, pumpkin, sesame and sunflower seeds. Like vegetables, seeds and nuts, particularly sesame and sunflower seeds, pistachios, pecans and almonds, are very high in magnesium, calcium and potassium.

However, nuts and seeds are very high in calories and can be difficult to digest, especially if roasted and salted. Therefore, eat them only in small to moderate amounts. Flax seed oil, one of the best sources of essential fatty acids, may be used as a butter substitute on vegetables, rice, potatoes, pasta and popcorn. Unlike butter, flax oil cannot be used for cooking, so add it for flavoring just before serving.

The oils in all seeds and nuts are very perishable, so avoid exposing them to light, heat and oxygen. Refrigerate all shelled seeds and nuts as well as their oils to prevent rancidity. Eating them raw and unsalted, removing the shells yourself, is healthiest. Seeds and nuts make a wonderful garnish on salads, vegetable dishes and casseroles. As your energy level improves, you can also eat them as a main source of protein in snacks and light meals.

Meat, Poultry and Fish

Eat meat only in small quantities—3 ounces or less per day—or avoid it altogether if you have moderate to severe anxiety. I recommend using meat mainly as a garnish and flavoring for casseroles, stir-fries and soups. When buying it, be sure to purchase only organic, range-fed animals for reduced exposure to pesticides, antibiotics and hormones.

Fish, particularly salmon, tuna, mackerel and trout, is a good source of antianxiety protein. Unlike other meat, fish contains linolenic acid, one of the beneficial fatty acids that help relax your mood as well as tense muscles, and is an excellent source of iodine and potassium. Other good sources of protein include grains, beans, raw seeds and nuts.

HOW TO SUBSTITUTE HEALTHY INGREDIENTS IN RECIPES

Making substitutions for high-stress ingredients allows you to use your favorite recipes, retain their flavor and taste and not compromise your health. You can also totally eliminate high-stress ingredients, for example, by making pizza with lots of vegetables but no cheese. Or you can cut down amounts of high-stress ingredients, for example, decreasing cow's milk cheese by one-half to two-thirds or sweetener by one-third to one-half.

Substitutes for Common High-Stress Ingredients

¾ cup sugar	½ cup honey
	¼ cup molasses
	½ cup maple syrup
	½ ounce barley malt
	1 cup apple butter
	2 cups apple juice
	Eliminate sweetener and add extra fruit and nuts to pastries
1 cup milk	1 cup soy, potato (DariFree), nut or grain milk
cheeses	Lower-fat cheeses, goat's or sheep's cheese; soy cheese in sandwiches, salads, pizzas, lasagnas and casseroles
1 tablespoon butter	1 tablespoon flax oil (must use raw, unheated; buy in health food stores)
½ teaspoon salt	1 tablespoon miso
	½ teaspoon potassium chloride salt substitute
	½ teaspoon Mrs. Dash, Spike
	½ teaspoon herbs (basil, tarragon, oregano)
	Powdered seaweeds (kelp or nori) to season vegetables, grains, salads. Add small amount of low-salt soy sauce or Bragg's Amino Acids to soups, casseroles, stir-fries at end of cooking process
1 ½ cups cocoa	1 cup powdered carob
1 square chocolate	¾ tablespoon powdered carob
1 tablespoon coffee	1 tablespoon decaffeinated coffee
	1 tablespoon Pero, Postum, Caffix or other grain-based coffee substitute
	Herbal teas; for morning pick-up, grate a few teaspoons of fresh ginger root into a pot of water, boil, steep and serve with honey
4 ounces wine	4 ounces light wine
8 ounces beer	8 ounces near beer
1 cup white flour	1 cup barley flour (pie crust)
	1 cup rice flour (cookies, cakes, breads)

VITAMINS, MINERALS, HERBS & ESSENTIAL FATTY ACIDS

Because poor or inadequate nutrition may play a major role in causing anxiety, optimal nutrition is an important facet of anxiety and stress treatment. A comprehensive nutritional program can help stabilize and relax your mood and promote optimal function of your immune system, glands and digestive tract. I have found it very difficult to relieve anxiety symptoms entirely when adequate nutritional support is lacking.

Most women have difficulty increasing their nutrient intake up to the levels needed for optimal healing using diet alone. Supplements can help correct the deficiency rapidly and completely. I must emphasize the importance of eating a good diet along with taking supplements; never take them while continuing poor dietary habits.

VITAMINS AND MINERALS

Many vitamins and minerals are useful in the treatment and prevention of anxiety. The supplements that provide the most symptom relief are discussed here.

Vitamin B Complex

This complex consists of 11 separate B vitamins that play an important role in healthy nervous system function. When one or more of these vitamins is deficient, symptoms of nerve impairment as well as anxiety, stress and fatigue can result. Conversely, adequate intake of these nutrients can help calm the mood and promote consistent energy levels.

Deficiencies of individual B vitamins increase anxiety and stress. Vitamin B6, for instance, affects moods through its important role in processing beneficial series-one prostaglandins. Lack of these relaxant hormones has been linked to PMS-related anxiety, menstrual cramps and stress-related problems like irritable bowel syndrome and migraine headaches. Using the birth control pill, a common treatment for PMS, menstrual cramps and irregularity, decreases vitamin B6 levels. Menopausal women on estrogen replacement therapy are also at risk of B6 deficiency. Anxiety symptoms can occur as a side effect of hormone use in both groups of women, in part because of B6 deficiency. Lack of B6 may also increase anxiety symptoms directly through the nervous system.

Women who are anxious and experiencing significant stress should eat foods high in B vitamins and use vitamin supplements. Because B vitamins are water soluble, the body cannot readily store them, so B vitamins must be consumed daily in the diet. Good sources of most B vitamins include brewer's yeast (which many women cannot digest readily), liver, chicken, salmon, shrimp, tuna, whole grain germ and bran, brown rice, beans, nuts, blackstrap molasses, sunflower seeds and such vegetables as asparagus, broccoli, cauliflower, green peas, leeks and sweet potatoes. Women following a vegan diet (a vegetarian diet with no dairy products or eggs) should take particular care to add supplemental vitamin B12 to their diets.

Vitamin C

This is an extremely important antistress nutrient that can help decrease the fatigue symptoms often accompanying excessive levels of anxiety. When the fight-or-flight pattern is activated in response to stress, adrenal gland hormones become depleted. Women with low vitamin C intake also tend to have elevated levels of histamine, a chemical that triggers allergy symptoms, which can cause emotional symptoms like anxiety. Larger amounts of vitamin C are needed when stress levels are high.

Vitamin C has also been tested, along with bioflavonoids, as a treatment for anemia caused by heavy menstrual bleeding—a common cause of fatigue and depression in teenagers and premenopausal women in their forties. One clinical study of vitamin C showed a reduction in bleeding in 87 percent of women taking supplements.

The best sources of vitamin C are fruits, including all citrus fruits, berries, cantaloupes, guavas and pineapples; most vegetables, but especially asparagus, Brussels sprouts, cabbage, collards, kale, potatoes, sweet peppers and tomatoes; and all types of liver, pheasant, quail and salmon. Since it is a water-soluble vitamin that is not stored in the body, women with anxiety should replenish their vitamin C supply daily through diet and supplements.

Bioflavonoids

Bioflavonoids often occur with vitamin C in fruits and vegetables. For example, they're found in grape skins, cherries, blackberries, blueberries and in the pulp and white rind of citrus fruits. They are also found in such foods as buckwheat and soybeans. Along with vitamin C, bioflavonoids strengthen the cells of small blood vessels and prevent anemia due to heavy menstrual bleeding, a common cause of fatigue and depression.

Bioflavonoids help normalize estrogen levels in a variety of gynecological conditions, thereby decreasing symptoms of anxiety that are linked to hormonal imbalances, particularly elevated estrogen levels. Because bioflavonoids are weakly estrogenic and antiestrogenic, they can lower excessive estrogen levels that trigger PMS and help relieve symptoms such as hot flashes, night sweats, anxiety, mood swings and insomnia in menopausal women grossly deficient in estrogen.

Vitamin E

Like bioflavonoids, vitamin E relieves symptoms of anxiety and mood swings triggered by the estrogen-progesterone imbalance experienced by women suffering from PMS and menopause. Women who find that conventional estrogen therapy worsens their anxiety symptoms (because drug doses do not match their body's needs) are potentially good candidates for vitamin E therapy. In women suffering from PMS, vitamin E helped alleviate anxiety, mood swings and food craving symptoms.

Vitamin E is a very important nutrient for women's health. The best natural sources of vitamin E are wheat germ, walnut, soy bean and other grain and seed oils, as well as almonds, asparagus, brown rice, cucumbers, haddock, herring, kale, lamb, mangoes, millet, peanuts and all types of liver. I recommend that women with menopause and PMS-related anxiety use between 400 to 2000 I.U. per day. Women with hypertension, diabetes or bleeding problems should start at 100 I.U. per day and increase the dosage slowly and carefully in consultation with their physician.

Magnesium

The body needs magnesium in order to produce ATP, the end product of the conversion of food to usable energy needed to fuel hundreds of thousands of chemical reactions. When magnesium is deficient, ATP production falls and the body forms lactic acid instead. Researchers have linked excessive lactic acid with anxiety and irritability symptoms. Deficiency of magnesium has also been found to cause signs of stress in the adrenal gland. This is noteworthy since the adrenal gland helps mediate physiological stress in the body.

Magnesium is also needed to produce the beneficial relaxant

prostaglandin hormones. Stimulating production of these hormones helps reduce the anxiety and mood swing symptoms of PMS, eating disorders and agoraphobia. Magnesium supplements can also benefit women with severe emotionally triggered anxiety and insomnia. When taken before bedtime, magnesium helps induce restful sleep.

Good food sources of magnesium include avocados, beans and peas, green leafy vegetables, raisins and dried figs, raw nuts and seeds, millet and other grains, tofu and a variety of meats, poultry and seafood.

Potassium

Like magnesium, potassium has a powerful enhancing effect on energy and vitality. It regulates the transfer of nutrients into the cells, aids proper transmission of electrochemical impulses and helps maintain nervous system function. The excessive use of coffee and alcohol (both of which can worsen anxiety and emotional stress symptoms) increases the loss of potassium through the urinary tract.

For women suffering from potassium loss, I recommend one to three 99-mg tablets or capsules per day to be used up to one week premenstrually. Potassium, however, should be avoided by women with kidney or cardiovascular disease, because a high level of potassium can cause an irregular heartbeat in women with these conditions. Since potassium can be irritating to the intestinal tract, it should be taken with meals. Potassium occurs in abundance in fruits, vegetables, beans and peas, seeds and nuts, starches and whole grains.

Calcium

The most abundant mineral in the body, calcium helps combat stress, nervous tension and anxiety. Like magnesium and potassium, calcium is essential for maintaining regular heartbeat and healthy transmission of nerve impulses. It may also help reduce blood pressure and regulate cholesterol levels. A calcium deficiency increases not only emotional irritability but also muscular irritability and cramps. Calcium can be taken at night along with magnesium to calm the mood and induce restful sleep. This is particularly helpful for women with menopause-related anxiety, mood swings and insomnia.

Many women do not consume the recommended daily allowance for calcium in their diet (800 mg for women during active reproductive years, 1200 mg after menopause), so a calcium supplement is useful. Good food sources of calcium include blackstrap molasses, green leafy vegetables, lamb, legumes, nuts and seeds, seafood, including salmon (with bones), tofu, whole grains and fruits, including berries, oranges, prunes and raisins.

Zinc

This mineral helps decrease anxiety by facilitating the action of B vitamins and creating proper blood sugar balance as well as healthy immune function, digestion and metabolism. Zinc is an essential trace mineral that helps reduce anxiety due to blood sugar imbalances and plays a role in normal carbohydrate digestion. Good food sources of zinc include wheat germ and other whole grains, apples, carrots, cabbage, chicken, legumes, onions, oysters, peaches, and soy products.

Chromium and Manganese

These two minerals are important in carbohydrate production and metabolism. Chromium helps keep the blood sugar level in balance so glucose (food) is properly used by the body. This avoids the extremes of too little glucose in the blood (hypoglycemia) or too much glucose (diabetes mellitus). By improving the intake of glucose into the cells, chromium helps the cells produce energy. Good sources of chromium include apples, bananas, brewer's yeast, chicken, molasses, oysters, potatoes, rye, spinach and whole wheat.

Manganese aids glucose metabolism and is also important in the digestion of food, especially proteins, and in the production of cholesterol and fatty acids. Good food sources of manganese include nuts and whole grains. Beans, leafy green vegetables, peas and seeds are also good sources when they are grown in soil containing manganese.

HERBAL RELIEF FOR CONDITIONS COEXISTING WITH ANXIETY

Many herbs can help relieve the causes and symptoms of stress, balance the diet and optimize nutritional intake.

• **Sedative and Relaxant Herbs:** By exerting a calming, restful effect on the central nervous system, the following herbs—balm, bay, catnip, celery, chamomile, hops, motherwort, passionflower, peppermint, skullcap, valerian, wild cherry and yarrow—relieve tight, tense muscles in the neck, shoulders, jaw and upper and lower back and promote restful sleep. If you suffer from menopause-related insomnia, for instance, make a strong sedative tea of hops or chamomile, using as many as two or three tea bags.

• **Blood Circulation Enhancers:** Ginger and ginkgo biloba improve circulation to tight, tense muscles; the two herbs can be effectively combined. To make ginger tea, grate a few teaspoons of fresh ginger root into a quart pot of water, boil, steep for 30 minutes and serve with a small amount of honey.

• **Herbs for Chronic Fatigue and Depression:** Anxiety and panic episodes can be exhausting to the body, stressing the endocrine and immune systems and other important systems. Women suffering from PMS, menopause, hypoglycemia and food allergies "roller coaster" between highs and lows during a single day. Women who use dandelion root, ginger, ginkgo biloba, oat straw and Siberian ginseng may note an increased ability to handle stress, as well as improved physical and mental capabilities.

• **Herbs for PMS and Menopause:** Many bioflavonoid-containing plants and herbs can be useful in the treatment of both PMS and menopause because they contain small amounts of the female hormones estrogen and progesterone. Anise, black cohosh, blue cohosh, citrus fruits, cherry, dong quai, false unicorn root, fennel, grape, hawthorn berry, red clover, sarsaparilla, unicorn root and wild yam root may be particularly useful for women who cannot or do not choose to use standard estrogen replacement therapy.

• **Herbal Digestants:** Fennel, garlic, ginger, papaya, papaya leaf and peppermint reduce symptoms of food intolerance such as bloating, abdominal cramps, diarrhea, constipation, fatigue, headache and mood swings by improving the digestive process.

• **Blood Sugar Stabilizers:** Siberian ginseng and gotu kola have been found to stabilize the blood sugar level, thereby reducing or eliminating the mood swings and symptoms of hypoglycemia.

ESSENTIAL FATTY ACIDS

Essential fatty acids (EFA) are an extremely important part of an antianxiety program. EFA—both linoleic (Omega 6 family) and linolenic acid (Omega 3 family)—are the raw materials from which beneficial hormone-like chemicals called prostaglandins are made. Prostaglandins have muscle-relaxant and blood-vessel-relaxant properties that can significantly reduce muscle cramps and tension. They also have a calming and relaxing effect on the emotions.

Because of their beneficial effects, EFA have been used in the treatment of anxiety, PMS, eating disorders and menopause.

EFA are not made by the body and must be supplied daily through food or supplements. The best food sources are raw flax seed and pumpkin seed oils (the raw seeds are good, too). Both must be absolutely fresh and unspoiled, so be sure to buy them in special opaque containers and keep them refrigerated. (You can also take them in capsule form.) Flax oil is my favorite because it has a wonderful flavor and can be used as a butter replacement on such foods as mashed potatoes, air-popped popcorn, steamed vegetables and bread. All essential oils should never be heated or used in cooking; just add them as a flavoring to foods that are already cooked.

Other good sources of linolenic acid are cold-water, high-fat fish such as salmon, tuna, rainbow trout, mackerel and eel. Good sources of linoleic acid include fresh raw sesame and sunflower seeds, wheat germ and corn, safflower, sesame seed, sunflower and wheat germ oils.

Some women may lack the ability to efficiently convert fatty acids to prostaglandins, which requires the presence of magnesium, vitamins B6 and C, niacin and zinc. This is especially true for women who eat a high-cholesterol diet and processed oils such as mayonnaise, use a great deal of alcohol or are diabetic. Other factors impeding prostaglandin production include emotional stress, allergies and eczema.

While the average healthy adult requires only 4 teaspoons per day of the essential oils, women with anxiety and stress symptoms who have a real deficiency may need up to 2 or 3 tablespoons per day until their symptoms improve. Occasionally, these oils may cause diarrhea; if this occurs, use only 1 teaspoon per day. Women with acne and very oily skin should use them cautiously. For optimal results, use these oils with vitamin E.

HOW TO USE VITAMINS, MINERALS AND HERBAL SUPPLEMENTS

Many women must use nutritional supplements to achieve high levels of essential nutrients. I recommend that women with anxiety take supplements cautiously. Start with one-quarter of the daily dose listed in the following formulas. Do not go to a higher dose unless you are sure you can tolerate it. Take all supplements with meals or a snack. If you have a digestive reaction, stop all supplements and start them again *one at a time* until you find the offending nutrient and eliminate it.

Supplementation for Anxiety, Panic, Food Addictions & Anxiety with Depression or Mitral Valve Prolapse

Vitamins and Minerals	Maximum Daily Dose
Beta-carotene	25,000 I.U.
B1, B2, B3, PABA	50–100 mg
B5, B6	50–200 mg
Choline, inositol	250–500 mg
B12	100 mcg
Folic acid, biotin	400 mcg
Vitamin C	2000–5000 mg
Vitamin D	400 I.U.
Vitamin E (d-alpha tocopherol acetate)	400–800 I.U.
Calcium aspartate	500–1000 mg
Magnesium aspartate	250–500 mg
Potassium aspartate	100–200 mg
Manganese	20 mg
Iron	18 mg
Zinc	15 mg
Copper	2 mg
Selenium	50 mcg
Chromium, iodine	150 mcg

Supplementation for Anxiety Related to PMS, Hypoglycemia & Hyperthyroidism

Vitamins and Minerals	Maximum Daily Dose
Beta-carotene	15,000 I.U.
Vitamin B complex:	
B1, B2, B3, B5, PABA	50 mg
B6	300 mcg
B12	50 mcg
Folic acid	200 mcg
Biotin	30 mcg
Choline bitartrate, inositol	500 mg
Vitamin C	1000 mg
Vitamin D	100 I.U.
Vitamin E	600 I.U.
Calcium	150 mg
Magnesium	300 mg
Iodine	150 mcg
Iron	15 mg
Copper	0.5 mg
Zinc	25 mg
Manganese	10 mg

Potassium	100 mg
Selenium	25 mcg
Chromium	100 mcg

Herbs (as capsules)	*Maximum Daily Dose*
Burdock, sarsaparilla	210 mg
Ginger	70 mg

Supplementation for Anxiety Related to Menopause

Women with mild to moderate symptoms can use the formula at half strength. Women with severe symptoms should use the full strength.

Vitamins and Minerals	*Maximum Daily Dose*
Beta-carotene	5000 I.U.
Vitamin A	5000 I.U.
Vitamin B complex:	
B1, B2, B3, B5, PABA	50 mg
B6	30 mg
B12	50 mcg
Folic acid	400 mcg
Biotin	200 mcg
Choline, inositol	50 mg
Vitamin C	1000 mg
·Vitamin D	400 I.U.
Vitamin E (d-alpha tocopherol acetate)	800 I.U.
Bioflavonoids	800 mg
Rutin	200 mg
Calcium citrate	1200 mg
Magnesium	320 mg
Iodine	150 mcg
Iron (ferrous fumarate)	27 mg
Copper	2 mg
Zinc	15 mg
Manganese	10 mg
Potassium aspartate	100 mg
Selenium	25 mcg
Chromium	100 mcg
Bromelain	100 mg
Papain	65 mg
Boron	3 mg

Herbs (as capsules)	*Maximum Daily Dose*
Anise, blessed thistle, black cohosh, fennel	100 mg

RELAXATION TECHNIQUES

Women with increased levels of anxiety often need to develop more effective ways of dealing with day-to-day stresses. By practicing self-help relaxation techniques, you can learn to manage stress more efficiently, make your thoughts peaceful and release tension, while you build self-esteem and self-confidence. Many patients report an increased sense of well-being by practicing the following techniques: focusing, meditation, grounding, releasing muscle tension and affirmations. Try them all, then decide which ones produce the greatest benefits for you and practice them regularly. You can also try taking a 20-minute warm bath, listening to classical music or nature sounds and having a massage either by a trained professional or your partner or by exchanging massages with a friend.

Exercise 1: Focusing
Select a small personal object that you like a lot, like a pin or a flower. Focus all your attention on it as you inhale and exhale slowly and deeply for one to two minutes. Try not to let any other thoughts or feelings enter your mind. If they do, return your attention to the object. At the end of the exercise you will probably feel calmer and any tension you had been feeling should be diminished.

Exercise 2: Meditation
- Sit or lie in a comfortable position. Close your eyes and breathe deeply and slowly, focusing all your attention on your breathing.
- Block out all other thoughts, feelings and sensations. If your attention wanders, bring it back to your breathing.
- As you inhale, say the word "peace;" as you exhale, say the word "calm." Draw out the pronunciation of the words so they last the entire breath. Repeating the words as you breathe will help you concentrate. Continue until you feel very relaxed.

Exercise 3: Oak Tree Meditation
- Sit in a comfortable position, your arms resting comfortably at your sides. Close your eyes and breathe deeply and slowly.
- Imagine that your body is a strong, solid oak tree with a wide, brown trunk. Imagine sturdy roots growing down from your legs, anchoring your body deep in the earth, so you can handle any stress.
- When upsetting thoughts or situations occur, visualize your body grounded like the oak tree. Feel strength and stability in your arms and legs. You feel confident, relaxed and able to handle any situation.

Exercise 4: Release of Muscle Tension and Anxiety
- Lie on your back in a comfortable position, your arms resting at your sides, palms down. Inhale and exhale slowly and deeply.
- Become aware of your feet, ankles and legs. Notice if these parts of your body have any muscle tension. If so, how does the tense part feel? Do you notice any strong feelings such as hurt, upset or anger there? Breathe into that place until you feel it relax, releasing any anxious feelings with your breath. Continue until the feelings begin to fade away.
- Continue the same process, moving up your body, first, into your hips, pelvis and lower back; then, into your abdomen and chest; and finally, into your head, neck, arms and hands.
- When you have released tension throughout your entire body, continue deep breathing for another minute or two. You should now feel lighter and more energized.
- **Alternative Exercise:** Clench your hands into fists, hold them tight for 15 seconds and relax the rest of your body. Visualized (imagine in your mind) your fists becoming tighter and tighter. Then relax your hands for 30 seconds and visualize a golden light flowing into your entire body, making all your muscles soft and pliable. Tense and relax the following parts of your body in this order: face, shoulders, back, stomach, pelvis, legs, feet and toes. When you're finished, imagine any remaining tension flowing out of your fingertips.

Exercise 5: Erasing Stress
- Sit or lie in a comfortable position. Breathe slowly and deeply. Visualize a situation, a person or even a belief (such as "I'm afraid of the dark," "I don't want to give a public speech" or "I'm afraid to go to the shopping mall") that causes you to feel anxious and fearful.
- You may see a specific person, an actual place or simply shapes and colors. Where do you see this stressful picture? Is it below

you, to the side or in front of you? How does it look? Is it big or little, dark or light, or does it have a specific color?

- Imagine that a large eraser (the kind used to erase chalk on a school blackboard) has just floated into your hand. Actually feel and see the eraser in your hand. Rub the eraser over the area with the stressful picture, so it fades, shrinks and finally disappears. When you can no longer see the stressful picture, continue to breathe deeply for another minute, inhaling and exhaling slowly and deeply.

Exercise 6: Positive Mind-Body Affirmations

Affirmations align your mind with your body in a positive way through the power of suggestion. While sitting in a comfortable position, repeat the following affirmations, saying ones that are important to you three times. Feel free to make up your own.

- I handle stress and tension appropriately and effectively.
- My mood is calm and relaxed.
- I can cope well and get on with my life during times of stress.
- I deserve to feel good right now.
- I feel grounded and fully present.
- I can effectively handle any situation that comes my way.
- I am thankful for all the positive things in my life.
- I am filled with energy, vitality and self-confidence.
- I am pleased with how I handle my emotional needs.
- I know how to manage my daily schedule to promote my emotional and physical well-being.
- I love myself and honor my body.
- I fill my mind with positive and self-nourishing thoughts.
- I am a wonderful and worthy person.
- I have total confidence in my ability to heal myself.
- I appreciate the positive people and situations that are currently in my life.

BREATHING EXERCISES

When you are in emotional distress, oxygen levels decrease as breathing becomes jagged, erratic and shallow. You may find yourself breathing too fast or you may even stop breathing altogether and hold your breath for periods of time without realizing it. None of these breathing patterns is healthful. The following therapeutic breathing exercises provide a way to break this pattern and help the mind and body return to peaceful equilibrium. They can help you even if you practice them only a few minutes each day.

Exercise 1: Deep Abdominal Breathing
- Lie flat on your back with your knees pulled up and your feet slightly apart. Breathe in and out through your nose. Inhale deeply, allowing your stomach to balloon out. Visualize your lungs filling up with air so your chest swells out.
- Imagine the air you breathe is filling your body with energy. Exhale deeply, letting your stomach and chest collapse.

Exercise 2: Peaceful, Slow Breathing
You can adapt deep abdominal breathing to reduce stress. Just imagine that the air you are breathing is filled with peace and calm and repeat the sequence until you feel relaxed.

Exercise 3: Grounding Breath
- Sit upright in a chair in a comfortable position, with your feet slightly apart. Breathe in and out through your nose. Inhale deeply, allowing your stomach to balloon out. Visualize your lungs filling up with air so your chest swells out. Hold your inhalation.
- See a large, thick cord running from the bottom of your buttocks to the center of the earth. Follow the cord all the way down and see it fastened securely to the earth's center. Run two smaller cords from the bottom of your feet down to the center of the earth.
- As you exhale, gently push your buttocks into the seat of your chair. Become aware of your buttocks, thighs, calves, ankles and feet. Feel their strength and solidity.
- Repeat this exercise several times until you feel fully grounded.

Exercise 4: Emotional Cleansing Breath
- Lie flat on your back with your knees pulled up and your feet slightly apart. Breathe in and out through your nose.
- Inhale deeply and see yourself enveloped in a soft white light. Breathe this cleansing light into every cell of your body to wash away fear, anger, anxiety and other negative feelings.
- As you exhale deeply, feel the light washing these emotions away.

- Repeat this exercise until you feel emotionally peaceful and clear.

Exercise 5: Depression-Release Breathing
- Sit upright in a chair. Cross your arms in front of your chest with your fingers touching the upper outer area of your chest. (Your wrists are crossed over your heart chakra, which is the energy center for emotions in traditional Asian healing models.) As you inhale, imagine golden light filling your heart center with a warm, loving feeling. As you exhale, breathe out depression and low spirits.
- As you inhale again, draw the golden light up through your neck and into your head, illuminating them with a soft, peaceful glow. Feel any negative thoughts dissolving as the light fills your brain.
- As you exhale, breathe the golden light out through the top of your head and see it form a shimmering cloud of energy around your entire body. Repeat the exercise 5 times.

PHYSICAL EXERCISE

Discharging physical and emotional tension through vigorous exercise directly and immediately reduces anxiety and stress. The long-term physiological benefits of exercise also build up your resistance to stress and promote beneficial psychological changes.

The many benefits of physical exercise include:

Improves resistance to and relief of anxiety episodes
- Reduces the fight-or-flight response
- Promotes cardiovascular resistance to stress
- Decreases skeletal muscle tension
- Reduces pent-up aggression and frustration
- Promotes a feeling of calm and peace

Improves brain function
- Promotes better oxygenation and blood circulation to the brain
- Increases output of beta endorphins (which create "runner's high")

- Improves concentration, problem solving, reaction time and short-term memory

Improves psychological functions
- Decreases anxiety and nervous tension
- Produces a sense of well-being and even elation
- Reduces depression
- Reduces insomnia
- Improves sense of mastery and self-confidence
- Promotes development of beneficial habits
- Helps decrease harmful addictive behavior

Improves physiological functions
- Stabilizes blood sugar level
- Reduces food craving
- Helps weight loss and maintenance
- Improves elimination through the bowels and kidneys
- Improves digestive functions
- Reduces blood pressure

BUILDING YOUR EXERCISE PROGRAM

If you are currently making the transition from a sedentary life-style to a regular exercise program, the first step is to evaluate your fitness level. It is important to know if you have any undiagnosed medical problems, like thyroid disease and hypoglycemia, that could affect your proper level of activity.

If you have not already done so, fill out the evaluation section questionnaires on your current exercise habits, patterns of muscle tension and symptoms of lack of physical fitness. If you have chronic muscle tension or feel out-of-breath after walking up a flight of stairs, you may actually have an underlying problem like anemia (low red blood cell count). I recommend you share your responses to the questionnaires with your health-care provider so she or he may discover any undiagnosed medical problem. Your physician should check your heart, lungs, pulse rate and other physical parameters to evaluate your exercise fitness. In addition, blood and urine tests may be ordered. Once you have received a clean bill of health or learn any health limitations, you can begin planning your exercise program.

The type of exercise regimen you choose can vary greatly depending on the goals you wish to accomplish. If your main goal is to relieve anxiety and improve your general health and well-being, then aerobic exercise is best. Aerobic exercise includes jogging, walking, bicycle riding, skiing, swimming, dancing, jumping rope and skating (see complete list in earlier section on evaluating symptoms). If you need to discharge pent-up anger, competitive sports such as handball, squash, racquetball, tennis and soccer may be best. If you find that playing games with other people helps reduce nervous tension, then try slower-paced sports like golf, croquet and bowling. If you like being outdoors, gardening can be very healing. Often, women may combine two or three types of exercises to meet a variety of goals.

Keep an exercise diary (described on page 16) during the first few months of developing a program. Using it provides a helpful organizational guide as well as a way to determine if your program is providing maximum anxiety-reducing benefits. If you skip a planned session, be sure to record the reason why, and record both positive and negative responses to your exercise sessions. Be sure to note if your anxiety, panic or stress symptoms increase, which can occur if you are pushing yourself too hard. In that case, reduce the length of time you are exercising and the intensity or type of activity.

Do not continue with an exercise program if it doesn't meet your ultimate goal: reduction of anxiety, stress and associated symptoms. Choose among a wide range of exercises and sports, and use your diary to help determine what mix of physical activities works best for you.

Before you begin your exercise program, read the following guidelines:

- Warm-ups such as stretching should always precede any athletic event. Wear loose, comfortable clothing. Evacuate your bowels or bladder before you begin. Working out before dinner is good since it helps diffuse tensions accumulated during the day.
- During the first week or two, build up your exercise level gradually, beginning with short sessions. For example, start out exercising every other day for 10 minutes. Then, increase sessions in 5-minute increments up to 30 and 60 minutes per session.
- Perform the exercise in a relaxed, unhurried manner. Set aside adequate time so you're not rushed. Anytime you feel anxiety, panic or excessive muscle tension, stop the exercise and reevaluate your pace.
- Avoid exercising when you are ill or during times of extreme stress. At such times the stress-reduction or breathing exercises may be more useful.
- Always rest for a few minutes after an exercise session.
- If you encounter mental obstacles to beginning and sticking with a regular exercise program, there are many ways to over-

come resistance: Make sure you exercise at the time of day that feels most natural and your schedule is least stressed. Be sure to choose exercises that you enjoy. Exercise in an attractive setting with a friend or support person; listening to mellow, relaxing music may help. Doing visualizations or saying affirmations will help prepare you positively for a routine.

YOGA

Yoga stretches promote a deep sense of peace and calm. Unlike fast-paced aerobic exercise, yoga actually slows down your pulse, heart rate and breathing, providing an oasis in which you can put aside your stress. Both the stress reduction effects and the physiological effects of yoga benefit all body systems. Always perform yoga stretches slowly and accompany them with deep, relaxed breathing.

The following yoga poses specifically reduce anxiety. Some work on the emotions, calming your mood and inducing serenity. Others help relieve the physical causes of stress, such as PMS and menopausal symptoms. Try all the exercises initially and see which ones produce the most beneficial results. Do yoga stretches three times a week or daily if they really help.

When doing yoga, it is important to focus your mind and concentrate on the positions. Pay close attention to the initial instructions. If you practice the stretch properly, you are much more likely to experience relief. First, read over the pose, visualizing it in your mind, then follow with the proper placement of the body. If you have any pain or discomfort, immediately reduce the amount of stretching until you can proceed without discomfort. If you strain a muscle, apply ice for 10 minutes. Use the ice pack two to three times a day for several days. If the pain persists, see your doctor.

Stretch 1: Child's Pose
- Sit on your heels. Bring your forehead to the floor, stretching the spine as far over your head as possible. Close your eyes. Hold for as long as it is comfortable.

Stretch 2: The Sponge

- Lie on your back with a rolled towel placed under your knees. Your arms are at your sides, palms up.
- Close your eyes and relax your whole body. Inhale slowly, breathing from your diaphragm. As you inhale, visualize the energy in the air being drawn into your entire body. Imagine your body is open like a sponge, drawing in energy to revitalize every cell.
- Exhale slowly and deeply, allowing every ounce of tension to drain from your body.

Stretch 3: Rock and Roll

- Lie on your back. Bend your knees, raising them to your chest. Interlock your fingers below your knees.
- Raise your head toward your knees and gently rock back and forth on your curved spine. Note the roundness of your back and shoulders. Keep your chin tucked in as you roll back, and avoid rolling back too far on your neck. Repeat 5 to 10 times. Rest briefly afterwards to enhance the stretch's benefit.

Stretch 4: The Locust

- Lie face down on the floor. Make fists with both hands and place them under your hips. This prevents compression of the lumbar spine while doing the exercise.
- Straighten your body and raise your right leg with an upward thrust as high as you can, keeping your hips on your fists. Hold for 5 to 20 seconds, if possible.
- Lower your leg to the original position. Repeat on the left side, then with both legs together. Repeat 10 times.

Stretch 5: The Bow

- Lie face down on the floor, arms at your sides. Slowly bend your legs at the knees and bring your feet up toward your buttocks.
- Reach back with your arms and carefully take hold of first one foot and then the other. Flex your feet so you can grasp them more easily.
- Inhale and raise your trunk from the floor as far as possible. Lift your head and elevate your knees off the floor.
- Squeeze your buttocks. Imagine your body looking like a gently curved bow. Hold for 10 to 15 seconds.
- Slowly release the posture, allow your chin to touch the floor and finally release your feet, slowly returning them to the floor. Return to your original position. Repeat 5 times.

Stretch 6: Side Rolls
- Lie on your back with your hands interlaced under your neck. As you inhale, bend and lift your right leg.
- Then exhale and roll on your left side, with your left knee touching the ground. As you do this, release a sigh.
- As you inhale, return to your original position. Repeat this 10 times, alternating sides. Then relax on your back for 1 minute.

ACUPRESSURE

Acupressure massage helps relieve both the emotional and the physical causes of anxiety. Based on an ancient Asian healing technique, it involves gentle finger pressure to specific points on the skin. Pressing specific points creates changes on two levels. Physically, acupressure affects muscle tension, blood circulation and other physiological matters. On another level, acupressure helps build the body's life energy, called *chi* (similar to electromagnetic energy). Health is thought to be a state in which sufficient chi is equally distributed throughout the body, energizing all the cells and tissues. Chi runs through the body in channels called meridians; disease occurs when the energy flow in a meridian is blocked. Meridian flow can be corrected by hand massage or stimulation with tiny needles (acupuncture). When the normal flow of energy is resumed, the body heals itself spontaneously.

Stimulation of acupressure points through finger pressure can be done by you or a friend following simple instructions. It is safe, painless and can be done without years of specialized training. Make sure your hands are clean and your nails trimmed to avoid bruising yourself. If your hands are cold, heat them with warm water.

Work on the side of the body that has the most discomfort. If both sides are equally uncomfortable, choose one. Working on one side seems to relieve symptoms on both sides.

Hold each point with steady, comfortable pressure with several fingers for 1 to 3 minutes. Apply pressure slowly with the tips of your fingers. If you feel resistance or tension, you may want to push a little harder. However, if your hand starts to feel tense or tired, lighten the pressure. If the acupressure point feels somewhat tender, it means the meridian is blocked. Tenderness should go away slowly during treatment. Some patients describe a very pleasant feeling of energy radiating out from this point into the body. Breathe gently while doing the exercises. You may massage the points once a day or more while you have symptoms.

Exercise 1: Use for Relief of Anxiety and Stress
Sit upright on a chair. Hold each step for 1 to 3 minutes.
- Left hand presses spot located in the slight depression on the top of the head. Right hand presses point directly between the eyebrows where the bridge of the nose meets the forehead.
- Right hand presses point in the center of your breastbone at the level of your heart. Your fingers will fit into the indentations in the bone.

Exercise 2: Use for Relief of Muscle Tension, Stress and Hypoglycemia
Hold each step 1 to 3 minutes.
- Roll up a towel lengthwise. Lie on your back and place the towel underneath your upper back between your shoulder blades. Relax in this position for 1 to 3 minutes.
- Now sit up. Left and right hands press points at the top of the shoulder blade, 1 to 2 inches away from the spine. The points may feel firm and resistant.
- Slide hands toward the top of the shoulder (where the neck meets the shoulder) and press.
- Move hands to the back of the neck, resting fingers on the muscles next to the spine, and press.
- Move hands underneath the base of the skull, 1 to 2 inches away from the spine (your fingers will feel a hollow), and press.

Exercise 3: Use for Relief of Insomnia
Sit comfortably and hold these points for 1 to 3 minutes.
- Left hand presses the point on the inside of the right ankle, located in the indention directly below the inner bone.
- Right hand presses the point in the indention below the right outer ankle.
- Repeat the point on the left foot.

Exercise 4: Relieves PMS and Menstrual-Related Anxiety
Sit on the floor and prop your back against a wall or a heavy piece of furniture. Hold each step 1 to 3 minutes. Alternative posi-

tion: Lie on the floor and put your lower legs over the seat of a chair.

- Press your right hand 1 inch above your waist on the muscle to the right side of the spine (the muscle will feel firm and ropelike), and keep it there throughout the exercise. Press your left hand behind the crease of your right knee.
- Move your left hand to the center of the back of your right calf and press. This is just below the fullest part of the calf.
- Move your left hand just below your ankle bone on the outside of the right heel and press.
- Move your left hand to the front and back of your right little toe at the nail and press.